Best Acne Treatment for Teens

An Unconventional System Which Will Cure Your Acne Fast & Naturally

By Trevor Thomas

Copyright © 2020
All rights reserved
ISBN: 9798605758297
Published by ZML Corp LLC

Disclaimer

This book is written for informational purposes only. The publisher and author shall have neither liability nor responsibility to any person or entity with respect to any loss or damage caused or alleged to be caused directly or indirectly by this book. This book has not been reviewed by a doctor or medical professional. You should talk and review this guide with your doctor and pharmacist before making any decisions.

This book is copyright 2020 with all rights reserved. It is illegal to copy, distribute, or create derivative works from this book in whole or in part or to contribute to the copying, distribution, or creating of derivative works of this book. Published by ZML Corp LLC. Written by Trevor Thomas.

The information contained on in this book is an opinion, and is for entertainment purposes only. You are responsible for your own behavior, and none of this book is to be considered legal or personal advice. And I expect you to abide by these rules. I regularly and actively search the internet for people who violate my copyrights. Now that we're finished with the disclaimer, let's learn about how to get rid of your acne.

Table of Contents

This Page Intentionally Left Blank

Chapter 1
My Background

Hi, my name is Trevor Thomas. I'm a former acne sufferer who has finally been able to put together a system that cured my acne. But before I tell you the system, let me give you a little background on my own struggle with acne.

I started getting acne when most people do, in my teen years. I remember getting my first pimple in 9th grade when I was 14... and that's where my fight with acne began.

A year later, by the age of 15, my acne started to get really bad. At this point I had pimples all over my face, as well as my chest and back. They were getting worse and worse each day, and my acne was starting to become cystic. Like most people, I first tried over the counter products. This included the face washes, the face wipes, the foams, the cleansers; I tried them all. They had absolutely no effect and literally did nothing. Then I decided I would try what the commercials told me, and I ordered Pro-Activ Solution. I followed the instructions and used the system exactly as described for two months. My acne did not improve one bit.

My skin was absolutely terrible. I was quite embarrassed about my acne, especially with so many people in my school with seemingly flawless skin. I decided to go to a dermatologist because enough was enough.

From the ages of 15-18, I was in and out of the dermatologist's office monthly. I went through 3 different doctors. I was put on every prescription acne pill and cream they make.

First I was put on a prescription lotion, Ziana. And while having mild results, my acne came right back. Then I was prescribed antibiotics with awesome results, but after just a few weeks, my acne came right back. For those whom have tried antibiotics, you may already know the issue, but what happens is the body starts becoming immune to them. Because of this issue, the dermatologist will put you on three different antibiotics and rotate them every so often in the attempt for the body to not become immune. This "treatment" only works for a little while, as the body ends up becoming immune to all three. And while I'm not a doctor, I feel this is one of the worst approaches a dermatologist can take with someone, as becoming immune to antibiotics can wreak havoc on you later in life if you actually need them. Not to mention the fact that when taken long term, antibiotics end up destroying not just the bad bacteria, but the good bacteria in your body as well.

Next I was prescribed STRONGER antibiotics with the same results. I felt so good acne free... for about 2 weeks. My acne ended up coming right back and even worse than before! My face was covered in pimples and blackheads. When doctors talk about severe acne, they are talking about the acne I had. On a scale of 1-10, by this time, I was about a 9.

My situation became desperate. I ordered anything online I could find. There were so many promises! So many creams! So many pills! But after literally thousands of dollars spent and every medication under the sun tried, I was still acne ridden... at 18 years old!

I just wanted to give up. What would you do at this point? When do you stop fighting? I decided I would live with my acne, hopefully it would go away by 25, and I would just deal with the fact I may have lots of scars on my face and trouble talking to women.

I was 18 at this time and went off to college, and yes, I still had acne. It kind of became like high school where people would stare at me or wouldn't talk to me because of my skin. So many people had beautiful skin. Why couldn't that be me?

But then something hit me. With all this great skin around, there has to be some people here with an acne solution. Why not just ask people what they do?

At this point I really didn't care what people thought of me. I was the most desperate person you've ever met when it came to finding a solution to get rid of my acne. So what if I talk to people. What do I have to lose? So that's what I did.

At first I started asking people who I knew for help. Though their advice was helpful, it wasn't perfect. After that, I started asking acquaintances such as people who sat next to me in class, people who lived in my dorm, people I ate with, etc. After a little while I just said, "screw it" and I literally started going up to random people with good skin and asking them what their secret was. I even went up to professors after class for advice!

Of course, many of these people told me things I already knew. The likes of "try Pro-Activ", "go to the dermatologist", and "wash your face". But even in a dark night sky, there are some shining stars. Some of the people I talked to actually had some wonderful advice! There were products I never heard of, techniques I had never tried, and research I didn't know existed.

So after talking to pretty much anyone and everyone at my college, I started trying their advice. Some things worked great... and some things were horrible. It took most of my college years, but after **A LOT** of trial and error, creams, lotions, pills, countless doctors' visits and thousands of dollars spent, I finally found a system that cured me of my acne and got my life back on track. And I'm confident it will work for you too!

The feeling of finally being acne free after so much heartache, depression, and the amount of time I spent with acne was incredible. I was literally speechless.

To this day I still use my system and will continue to use it for as long as I have acne. I now know the feeling of being acne free, and it feels great. My confidence is alive. I'm back to being myself. I want you to experience what I feel. So go on and read the rest of this book, try out this system for yourself, and experience the joy of finally being acne free! Good luck my friend.

Chapter 2
Diet

In this chapter, I want to go over some of the myths and misconceptions regarding acne, and why much of the information that we're told about acne is not actually true. Some of this information you may already know, but likely a lot of it will be new to you. After reading, I encourage you to do your own research and then try out my advice.

One of the biggest myths I've been told regarding acne, and which many dermatologists subscribe to, is diet has no effect on acne. They say acne is just a part of puberty, or that some people are just more prone to acne than others. I remember during my countless dermatology visits, not once did any of the three dermatologists mention diet. All they did was prescribe me creams and pills. I'm here to tell you diet is the number one factor that causes acne and countless research studies, as well as my own experience, are here to prove it!

There was a flawed study from the 1960's that concluded that diet had no effect on acne. This study has been taught in textbooks, patient brochures and medical literature. Many dermatologists still subscribe to this, as it is the primary philosophy taught about acne in medical school. During the study, researchers gave participants a chocolate bar to eat, and evaluated them over a four week period. The study concluded the chocolate bar did not have an effect on patient's acne, and thus diet has no effect on acne. Can you see the obvious flaws associated with this study?

In American medical schools, MD's (allopathic doctors) are taught to treat you with pharmaceuticals. Very little of the education they receive involves diet and preventing the disorder, but instead revolves around symptoms and fixing the disorder that has already happened. Many medical schools are supported by or have some type of connection to big pharmaceutical companies. The approach of "treat the symptom" leads to much bigger profits for pharmaceutical companies because you'll end up taking the medication for much longer, as your symptoms will keep coming back. This is because you're not fixing the root of the problem.

Another thing to consider is pharmaceutical companies make money from their medicine. And if pharmaceutical companies cannot patent a medicine, another company can come in, steal the idea, and then they end up losing money from all their hard work and research. This means anything they can't patent, they are not going to spend money researching. This includes vitamins, diets, supplements, etc. Anything "natural" you could do on your own without them. Thus they don't teach it to doctors at medical schools, the doctors don't bring it up with you at your visits, and you don't end up hearing about it.

Acne is just one of the many disorders that pharmaceutical companies make billions from. Obviously pharmaceutical drugs have their place in medicine and have added many benefits to our lives, but for some disorders they are not the answer.

When it comes to the human body, everyone is different. If you take a look around your school or work place, you'll see some people can eat anything they want and don't gain an ounce of weight. Well it's the same way with acne. Some people can eat anything they want and yet still have flawless skin. They don't have one pimple on their face and may have never had acne. These people are the exception. The majority of people do get acne in their teenage years and for many, including myself, it remains a problem well into adulthood. And the main reason they get it is because of their diet.

<u>Glycemic Index</u>

The main culprit of acne is the western style diet that has taken over the world in recent years. The diet includes high carb, high sugar, high glycemic index foods that spike your blood sugar and dramatically increase your prevalence of acne. You see, it's the spike in blood sugar caused by high glycemic index foods that is the main cause of acne for many sufferers.

When your blood sugar spikes, it causes inflammation in your body. Inflammation and acne are known to have a direct correlation. So the more foods you ingest that spike your blood sugar, the more inflammation you develop, and the more acne you get. The amount your blood sugar spikes, which in turn is the amount of inflammation produced in your body, is demonstrated in the glycemic index.

The glycemic index is a number scale that ranges from 0-100. Foods that spike your blood sugar, which include sugary, high carb foods, are towards the upper end (> 55), and these are foods that acne sufferers should avoid. Examples of high glycemic index foods include soda (63), ice cream (62), white bread (73), and pure glucose (100). Foods on the lower end of the spectrum (< 55) cause minimal spikes in blood sugar, and are the foods that acne sufferers should stick to eating. Examples of these foods include black beans (30), carrots (39), and unbreaded meat. More information can be found regarding the glycemic index at the websites below:

Harvard Health
bit.ly/gindex1

MayoClinic
bit.ly/gindex2

University of Sydney
bit.ly/gindex3

There are also many great books available that can teach you more about the glycemic index as well. Examples include "The GI Diet" by Rick Gallop and "The Glycemic Load Diet" by Rob Thompson.

An example I want to provide you that really proves the point that diet is so closely linked to acne is an island off the coast of Papa New Guinea called Kitava. On this island are a group of indigenous people whose diets differ dramatically from the typical western diet found around the world. Their diet consists mostly of fruit, vegetables and fish; no soda, no fruit roll ups, no Wonder bread. Their diet is considered a low glycemic index diet. Acne is completely unheard of on this island, even in teenagers. Diabetes, cardiovascular diseases and dementia are other disorders which do not exist on this island. How can this be if acne happens to "everyone" and is just a result of "hormones"? The answer is it isn't.

The explanation in this book is just a short summary of the glycemic index. I encourage you to visit the websites above, read the books I have listed, and do your own research on the glycemic index. This will give you a better understanding of how it works, as well as show you a more complete list of the foods you can eat, as well as the ones you should stay away from.

Now let's dive into some of the main foods that can cause problems for acne.

Sugar

If I could give you just one thing to eliminate from your diet that would allow you to see dramatic improvements in your acne within days, it's sugar. Sugar is your absolute worst enemy when it comes to acne. This is because of the inflammation is causes in your body.

You may not realize it, but there are so many products that contain sugar that you may not even be aware of. I highly encourage you to watch a documentary on Netflix called "Fed Up". It provides further evidence to support this book, and highlights how sugar is hidden in so many foods and the issues it causes to our health.

Sugar is not just contained in known foods like soda or candy, but also hidden in other foods like bread. White bread, and similar white products (e.x. white pasta, crackers) are simple carbohydrates. After being eaten, these foods quickly turn into sugar in the body, producing the same acne causing inflammation as soda or candy.

For the most part, the only food that contains sugar that is okay to eat is fruit. This is because fruit contains fiber which offsets the blood sugar spike associated with most sugary foods. Some fruits are better than others, and this relates back to the glycemic index talked about before.

Soda, fruit snacks, sweetened apple sauce, and many other products you may currently be eating are pure sugar and show a direct link to acne. Fruit juice is not okay either. The issue with fruit juice is all the fiber is taken out, and you are only getting the sugar and taste from the fruit. This includes orange juice, apple juice, cranberry juice, etc. and even the "healthy" juices like the "Naked" juices made by Pepsi. They are all touted as "healthy", however you're no better off chugging a soda, as they both contain the same amount of sugar and fiber.

And sugar is sugar is sugar. You may see products like "Sugar in the Raw", "Organic Sugar", or hear how high fructose corn syrup is worse than sugar. It's all the same and all treated as your body as sugar. You could drink a cup of soda or a cup of orange juice; the sugar in both of these are treated by the body as the same and cause the same inflammation.

Local smoothie shops like "Smoothie King" are guilty of the same thing. Some of their smoothies pack over 4x the recommended daily allowance of sugar by the American Heart Association. A 40oz "Apple Kiwi Kale" smoothie from Smoothie King has 131 grams of sugar and just five grams of fiber! Compare this to an apple that has the same amount of fiber with just 19 grams of sugar. A good rule of thumb is to look at the fiber in the food or drink you're ingesting. You can subtract the amount of fiber by the amount of sugar in it to get a gauge of how much sugar you're actually consuming.

My main problem, which you may suffer from too, was soda. I drank soda from about five years old till I turned 22, which is when I started changing my diet. I would drink soda every day, well over 40oz on average. This included energy drinks like Monster, which are essentially soda with more caffeine and some B-vitamins. Soda is all around us and a big part of the American diet. Go to any restaurant and your drink choices are basically soda or water. I would drink soda with almost every meal, and I didn't even give it a second thought. I ended up giving up soda when I changed my diet and just this one small change alone dramatically improved my acne in just days! It was like a light switch. If you struggle with a slight soda addiction, I find flavored seltzer water is a great alternative. This is the seltzer water that contains carbonated water and natural flavors such as LaCroix sparkling water. This is NOT the seltzer water that contains artificial sweeteners like aspartame or sucralose.

Diet drinks, such as diet coke, diet fruit juice and some seltzer waters are NOT a viable alternative to their sugary counterparts, and may actually be worse. Research finds that the sugar substitutes in these drinks, which include sucralose and aspartame, are recognized by the body the same as sugar and spike blood sugar in the same way. Thus, they cause the same problems for acne sufferers as sugary drinks, not to mention the other health issues that have been attributed to artificial sweeteners, particularly aspartame.

So if you're an avid fan of any of the drinks I've mentioned which include soda, energy drinks, fruit juice, etc., the first thing you can do is try cutting them out, or cut back drastically. Replace these sugary drinks with either water or seltzer water. If you are a fan of energy drinks, try drinking coffee or the energy shots like "5 Hour Energy" instead. These energy shots do contain artificial sweeteners, however at only 2 ounces in size, the amount is quite small. And two packets of sugar in your coffee, which should satisfy those with a sweet tooth, contains just 8 grams of sugar, compared to 54 grams of sugar in a 16 ounce Monster energy drink. Another option is to take caffeine pills when you're feeling tired and need some caffeine. A pack of 90 caffeine pills at Walmart go for about $4. One caffeine pill contains no sugar, and has the same amount of caffeine as a small cup of Starbucks coffee (200mg).

If you are an avid drinker of sugary drinks, just this one tip alone will provide dramatic results for your acne.

<u>Water</u>

While cutting out sugary drinks is a good first step, you need to replace those drinks with something. Water, or seltzer water with natural flavors, is really the only thing you should be drinking.

The body is made up of about 60% water. And while your body has numerous uses for water, it's especially important for the skin. Think of your body as a long set up pipes that sometimes get clogged. Throughout the day, toxins can build up in our bodies from the foods we eat. These toxins can cause and exacerbate acne. Water can flush out these pipes (your body), removing the toxins and thus helping to prevent acne.

You should be drinking at least 64 ounces of water a day, however the more the better. Some people drink a gallon of water a day. It may seem like a lot, but you easily drink this much in a day already, just probably through soda or other sugary drinks. Get yourself a refillable, dishwasher safe water bottle and start using it every day. Bring it in the car with you, bring it to class, bring it to work. Wherever you are, make sure to have some water with you. Replacing all the sugary drinks with water will dramatically improve your skin for the better.

<u>Dairy</u>

As everyone's body is different, dairy may not be a big factor for all, however it's worth seeing if giving up dairy has an effect on your skin. While you may not be diagnosed as lactose intolerant, your body may still present problems when dairy is eaten, and acne would be one of them.

Dairy is a known inflammatory and thus can be a cause of acne in some people's diet. I would suggest giving up dairy for a few weeks and see what kind of effect it has on your skin. This would include milk, cheese, Cheetos, etc. Anything that contains milk products should be avoided. If your skin improves, you found a trigger for your acne. If not, move on and try other ideas discussed in this book.

Many seemingly dairy free products may actually contain dairy, so be sure to read labels. Examples would include crackers, salad dressings, and potato chips.

Chapter 3
External Products

While diet is the main factor when it comes to controlling your acne, there are some external products that can also be quite helpful.

Acne Light

Recently it has been found that certain wavelengths of light can have great benefits for your skin, and acne in particular. At first, these light treatments were only available in dermatologist offices and quite expensive. However, as with any new product, the cost has come down dramatically and there are now at home products acne sufferers can use. One product I recommend, which I use personally, is the Neutrogena Acne Mask.

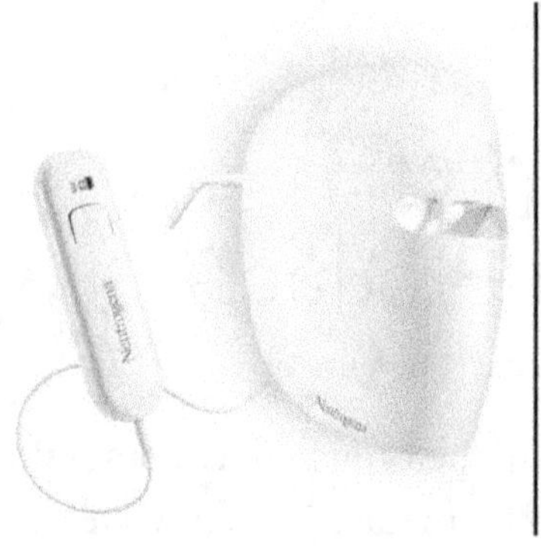 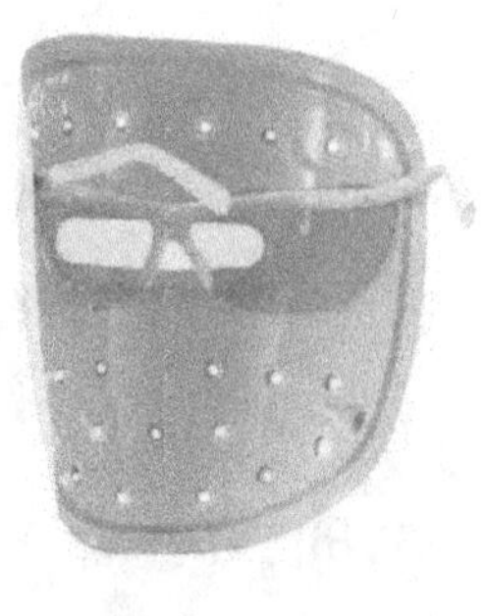

This light mask is chemical free, drug free, UV free, and clinically proven to improve acne! It retails for $20-$30 at most major retailers. Here is a shortened link which will take you to the Amazon page of this product: **fastlink.xyz/mask**

Light is measured in a spectrum, with visible light being between 400 – 700 nanometers. What scientists have found is certain wavelengths of light have beneficial effects on the skin. The acne light above uses LED's to generate two wavelengths of light. The first light is a blue 414 nanometer light that kills p. acne bacterium, the bacteria that causes acne. The second light is a red 610 nanometer light that promotes healing of the skin. Both of these wavelengths of light are found in the sun's rays, however you can't sit in front of the sun, as there would be more problems than benefits from that treatment option.

What's great about this light is it's effective for almost everyone, unlike some other treatments which are hit or miss. In a 12 week clinical trial, 98% of patients who used this light saw improvement in their skin.

There is no ultraviolet (UV) light in this mask, as it uses LED lights. So there is no risk associated with burning your skin, hurting your eyes, or radiation. However the light is quite bright, so I personally cut out the nose piece on my mask, and use tanning goggles. While not required, I find the experience more tolerable as the lights are extremely bright.

How it works is you put on the mask and wear it for ten minutes. I usually just close my eyes and listen to music while I wear it. The instructions recommend using it three times a week, however the more the better. I try to use it four to five times a week. This mask doesn't just treat existing acne, but prevents acne from forming, which is why using it consistently is key to its effectiveness.

The mask runs on AA batteries and can be used thirty times. Then an additional "activator" needs to be purchased to use it again. This activator connects to the end of mask, and is easily detached/reattached to start using again. If you search on the internet, there's a way to jerry-rig the mask to be able to use it an unlimited amount of times without having to buy additional "activators". It involves buying an on/off switch, and connecting it with wire to the inside of the battery compartment. If you're tech savvy, this may be something you want to look into, as it can save you some money.

Note: I've found many tanning salons and fitness facilities (Planet Fitness in particular) are now offering full body versions of these lights to help with people's skin. So you may want to call some places in your area and see if they offer this service. This would be particularly helpful if you have body acne. It will get a little expensive though, and you most likely won't be able to use it as much as an at home face light, but just something to consider.

Life Link Metazene 5% Gel

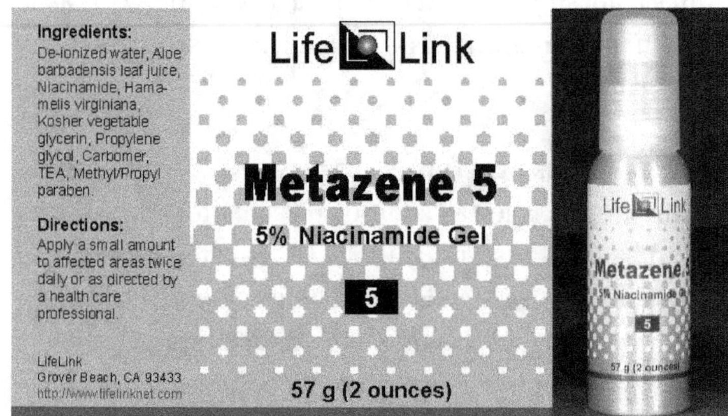

I found this gel out of pure luck and I'm so happy I did. Like many of you reading this book right now, I had never heard about this gel as it's made by small company and of course, my dermatologist did not tell me about it. I was at a coffee shop, acne ridden, and I went up to a random guy drinking his coffee. I asked him if he knew any good products for acne and he told me about this one. The gel is called Metazene and it is made by a small company called "Life Link". The main ingredient in the gel is Niacinamide, which is a B-Vitamin that helps with skin conditions. This gel takes it one step further and puts it in topical form.

Researchers at a New York state university found this gel had better results than clindamycin, which is a powerful antibiotic dermatologists prescribe to treat acne. Not only that, it doesn't produce the negative side effects that many other topical treatments can cause like dry, red or flaky skin.

This gel contains three substances that fight against acne:

- Niacinamide (Main Ingredient)
- Hamamelis Extract
- Aloe

It comes in a 2-ounce bottle with a dispensing pump that dispenses a measured amount with the press of a finger. Niacinamide has a scientifically documented track record as an anti-acne treatment which includes:

- Suppressing inflammation, the cause of much of the skin disruption seen in acne.

- Reducing sebum production in hair follicles, limiting its availability to bacteria which thrive in it.

- Improving the skin's water barrier function, which is impaired in acne-prone skin.

And not only does it help with acne, a clinical trial in 2005 concluded that this gel helps with aging too! They said it resulted in "reductions in fine lines and wrinkles, hyperpigmented spots, red blotchiness, skin sallowness, and improved elasticity."

Here is a shortened link to the product page:

fastlink.xyz/metazene

Chapter 4
Supplements

Most of what causes acne comes from inside the body, which is why supplements can be such a big help for acne sufferers. While diet is the most important aspect of fixing your acne and should be the main method used, supplements do have their place and can be very beneficial in your fight against acne.

As stated before, everyone is different. The human body is quite interesting in how it works. Ask any doctor or pharmacist, and they'll tell you patients who have had tremendous results with a medication, and yet other patients who received no benefit from it at all. For certain medical conditions, patients have to try a few different medications before finding one that works well for them. Everyone's body is different and reacts differently to pharmaceuticals.

It's the same with supplements. One of these supplements may work great for you, one may do nothing. I recommend starting one at a time with these supplements and seeing what works for you. Give it a few weeks and re-evaluate your skin. If it works, continue taking it. If not, move on and try the next one. Unfortunately the human body does require some trial and error.

When buying supplements, make sure to stick to a reputable brand. Unfortunately they are not regulated like pharmaceuticals, and companies have been caught in the past selling supplements that don't actually contain the listed ingredients. One brand in particular guilty of this was Spring Valley, which was investigated by the New York attorney general in 2015.

Supplements that are "USP" certified are considered reputable, as this means a 3rd party has come in to examine them for purity. Unfortunately not many companies get USP certifications for their supplements, but that doesn't necessary mean they aren't pure. There is a website called ConsumerLab.com which independently tests supplements for purity. At $3 a month, it may be worth it to subscribe if you plan on using supplements to help your skin. I will be recommending supplements in this book from brands that have worked well for me, however feel free to use whatever brand you would like.

There are two types of supplements: fat soluble and water soluble. Fat soluble supplements (e.x. Vitamin

A, Vitamin E), can build up in your body if you take too high of a dose over a long period of time, and can have damaging effects on the liver. Water soluble supplements (e.x. Vitamin B, Vitamin C) do not build up in your body, as excess is urinated out. While you technically can still overdose on water soluble vitamins, the amount needed for this to happen is usually extremely high. Just understand while the risks are low, there are still risks to supplements if you don't follow the directions on the bottle or go above max recommended daily doses.

Before trying any supplements, be sure to talk with your doctor and pharmacist to get their professional medical advice. You also want to start slowly, and be sure not to go over the tolerable upper intake limit (UL) which can be found on WebMD. This is the amount that can be safely taken each day without causing problematic side effects.

Disclaimer I am not a medical doctor and not able to give medical advice. Talk with your doctor and pharmacist before trying any supplements to be sure they will have no ill-effects on yourself, health conditions you have, or interact with any medications you are taking. The information below is for informational purposes only.

Zinc

Research has shown Zinc is as effective as oral antibiotics for treating acne. There seems to be a correlation with the severity of a patient's acne and their blood levels of zinc. People with acne typically have about 24% lower zinc levels than non-acne sufferers. While scientists are not sure of the exact reasons behind why zinc helps with acne, they do know a few things:

- Zinc is a powerful antioxidant and some studies show taking antioxidants can help reduce acne.

- In test tube studies, zinc killed acne causing bacteria. And unlike antibiotics, the bacteria cannot become resistant to zinc.

- Zinc is an anti-inflammatory.

If you have not tried Zinc, this is an extremely beneficial supplement. If there is just one supplement you try from this book, it should be zinc.

There are different types of zinc (e.x. zinc oxide, zinc gluconate), and your body is able to absorb certain forms of zinc better than others. The best type of zinc you can take is called OptiZinc. It is the most absorbable form of zinc for your body, and has been shown to provide the best results for acne sufferers. I personally use the supplement "NOW L-OptiZinc" which can be found here: **fastlink.xyz/zinc**

NAC

A study came out in 2012 that showed a correlation between antioxidant levels and patients with acne. I'm sure you've heard the term "antioxidants" before, as it's a popular buzz word. Antioxidants are commonly found in fruits and vegetables, and help prevent or stop damage to cells caused by oxidants.

For some reason, people with acne seemed to have lower antioxidant levels in their body than non-acne sufferers. Researchers noticed this correlation and decided to conduct a study. Participants in the study were split up into groups, and each group was given a different antioxidant to take. Results were recorded over several weeks until the study concluded. N-acetyl cysteine, or NAC for short, seemed to be one of the most effective antioxidants they used. The study found NAC was able to reduce acne in patients by 50%. Now Foods has an excellent version of this supplement which can be found here: **fastlink.xyz/nac**

Vitamins A and E

In a study from 2006 in "Clinical and Experimental Dermatology", participants with acne where found to have significantly lower blood levels of vitamins A and E than non-acne sufferers. The study concluded that low levels of vitamin A and E show a strong correlation to causing acne. While the study did not conduct clinical trials, many acne sufferers on forums have experimented with these vitamins, and experienced significant results.

Vitamins A and E are fat soluble vitamins. USP certified versions of both from Nature Made can be found at the links below:

Vitamin A – **fastlink.xyz/a**
Vitamin E – **fastlink.xyz/e**

Vitamin D

Vitamin D is thought to reduce the growth of cells that produce sebum, reducing the amount of oil your skin produces and thus reducing acne.

In 2016, a study conducted in South Korea compared vitamin D levels of people with acne to those with clear skin. Results found that about half of the acne sufferers were deficient in vitamin D. They conducted a trial and found that treatment with vitamin D resulted in a 35% reduction in acne after two months.

Vitamin D is a fat soluble vitamin. A USP certified version from Nature Made can be found here: **fastlink.xyz/d**

L-Lysine

L-lysine is an amino acid, and one that your body is incapable of producing on its own. Different amino acids have different functions. L-lysine is used by the body in collagen formation and skin tissue repair. It also is said to help with viral infections by removing certain bacteria in the body. Propionibacterium acnes, the bacteria that causes acne, is one of the bacteria l-lysine is said to remove. This is the main reason l-lysine is thought to be so beneficial for people with acne. NOW Foods has a version of L-Lysine which can be found here: **fastlink.xyz/lysine**

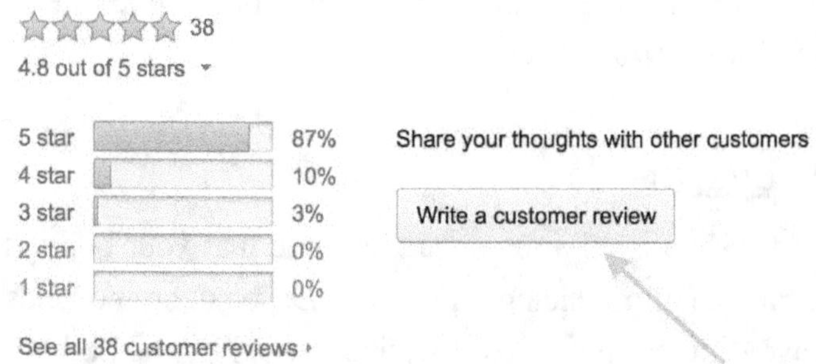

If you are enjoying this book, could you please leave a review on Amazon? It would be greatly appreciated and allow me to come out with more informative books in the future. A shortened link to the review page is below:

fastlink.xyz/acne

Chapter 5
The System

It's time to get rid of your acne! Depending on the severity of your acne and how you respond to the different treatment options, you may not have to do everything laid out in the instructions below. It's possible just one of these treatment options will completely clear your acne. Everyone is different.

If your acne is more severe, it is likely you will need to include more of the products I have suggested in your treatment plan, as well as be a little more patient with the amount of time your acne takes to completely disappear. Below is the system to use to eliminate your acne.

Instructions:

1. Apply the Metazene gel twice a day; once in the morning and once at night.

2. Use the acne light at least 3 times a week. If you can, build it into a routine and use it every day. It's just ten minutes and it works so well!

3. Drink Water! Drink at least 64 ounces of water a day. Cut out all the sugary drinks and just drink water or seltzer water instead. I understand it may not be fun, but your skin will thank you!

4. Stick to a low glycemic index diet as described in chapter two.

5. Try out one supplement at a time and take the supplement daily, being sure to be consistent. Wait at least 2-3 weeks before you decide if a supplement is working for you, as results do take time to show. I recommend starting with Zinc.

After following the instructions described above, you will start noticing results immediately in your skin. And soon, you're acne will completely go away.

Now I imagine some of the products, supplements, or ideas mentioned in this book may be new to you. For that reason, don't take my word for it, do your own research! You'll find, just as I did, everything I describe has great results for getting rid of your acne and providing clear skin.

Conclusion

I hope I was able to help you in your fight against acne and you learned new information from this book. If you incorporate all the advice I have given you and strictly follow this system, you will start noticing results immediately and soon be completely acne free.

I want to mention that everything I have talked about in this book is real. Everything I have proclaimed about myself is true. I was acne ridden. I did try everything I said I did. I really have spent thousands of dollars on acne products and at dermatologist offices. And after all was said and done, this treatment plan is the only thing that has ever been truly effective for me. It will work for you too!

Make sure to do your own research on the information I laid out for you in this book. The more you understand about the condition of acne, and why the treatments laid out in this book work, the better you will be able to treat your own acne.